Hiatal Hernia Syndrome Guide for Beginners

Preventive Measures of Hiatal Hernia Syndrome

By

Lachlan Hubert

Table of Contents

CHAPTER 1

Introduction

A comprehensive understanding of hiatal hernia syndrome begins with a closer examination of its fundamental aspects, including its definition, the underlying causes, and the common symptoms experienced by individuals afflicted with this condition. This introductory section will lay the foundation for the subsequent exploration of hiatal hernia syndrome.

1.1 What is Hiatal Hernia Syndrome?

Hiatal hernia syndrome is a medical condition that affects the upper gastrointestinal tract and occurs when a portion of the stomach protrudes into the chest cavity through an opening in the diaphragm known as the esophageal hiatus. The diaphragm, a crucial muscular structure separating the chest cavity from the abdominal cavity, plays a pivotal role in respiration. However, in cases of hiatal hernia syndrome, the hiatus becomes enlarged or weakened, allowing the stomach to push through into the thoracic region, leading to various symptoms and potential complications.

Hiatal hernias are classified into several types, the most common being the sliding hiatal hernia, where the junction of the esophagus and stomach slides into the chest. Paraesophageal hiatal hernias are less common but more concerning, as they involve a portion of the stomach alongside the esophagus, potentially leading to strangulation and serious complications. Mixed hiatal hernias encompass characteristics of both sliding and paraesophageal hernias.

Understanding hiatal hernia syndrome also requires consideration of its prevalence. While the exact number of affected individuals varies, it is estimated that hiatal hernias are relatively common, with older adults and individuals with risk factors being more susceptible. Though not always symptomatic, hiatal hernia syndrome can lead to discomfort and complications, necessitating appropriate diagnosis and management.

1.2 Causes and Risk Factors

The causes of hiatal hernia syndrome are multifactorial, with various risk factors contributing to its development. Some of the prominent causes and risk factors include:

- **Aging:** Hiatal hernias tend to be more common among older adults due to natural weakening of the diaphragm and supporting structures over time.

- **Obesity:** Excess body weight can exert pressure on the abdominal region, increasing the risk of hiatal hernia development.

- **Inherited Factors:** There is evidence to suggest a genetic component in the development of hiatal hernias, with a family history of the condition potentially increasing one's risk.

- **Trauma:** Abdominal injuries or surgeries can weaken the diaphragm, making herniation more likely.

- **Smoking:** Smoking is associated with chronic coughing and increased abdominal pressure, both of which can contribute to hiatal hernia development.

- **Heavy Lifting:** Frequent heavy lifting, especially when done with improper technique, can strain the diaphragm and raise the risk of herniation.

- **Pregnancy:** The hormonal changes and pressure exerted

by a growing fetus can lead to hiatal hernias in pregnant individuals.

- **Chronic Constipation:** Straining during bowel movements, common in cases of chronic constipation, can contribute to herniation.

Understanding the causes and risk factors is essential for both prevention and early detection of hiatal hernia syndrome. Identifying and addressing these underlying factors can help reduce the risk of hernia development and associated complications.

1.3 Common Symptoms

Hiatal hernia syndrome is often characterized by a range of symptoms that can vary in intensity and presentation. Some of the most common symptoms associated with hiatal hernias include:

- **Heartburn:** Individuals with hiatal hernias are prone to gastroesophageal reflux disease (GERD), leading to heartburn—a burning sensation in the chest, often after meals.

- **Regurgitation:** Regurgitation occurs when stomach contents flow back into the esophagus or even the mouth, leading to an unpleasant taste.

- **Dysphagia:** Difficulty swallowing is another common symptom, particularly when the hernia compresses the esophagus.

- **Chest Pain:** The chest pain experienced by those with

hiatal hernias can be similar to heart-related chest pain (angina) and may be mistaken for a heart issue.

- **Belching and Hiccups:** Frequent belching, hiccups, or an increased sensation of bloating may occur.

- **Nausea and Vomiting:** Some individuals experience nausea and vomiting, especially after large meals.

- **Respiratory Symptoms:** Severe hiatal hernias can cause respiratory symptoms, such as shortness of breath and a chronic cough.

- **Unintended Weight Loss:** In cases of significant complications, such as strangulation of the hernia, unintended weight loss may occur.

Understanding these common symptoms is crucial for the early recognition and diagnosis of hiatal hernia syndrome. Timely intervention and management can help improve the quality of life for affected individuals and prevent potential complications.

CHAPTER 2

Types of Hiatal Hernias

Hiatal hernias are classified into several types based on their specific characteristics and the way in which they affect the anatomy of the upper gastrointestinal tract. Each type of hiatal hernia presents unique challenges and potential complications.

2.1 Sliding Hiatal Hernia

A sliding hiatal hernia, also known as a type I hiatal hernia, is the most common form of hiatal hernia. In a sliding hiatal hernia, a portion of the stomach and the junction of the esophagus and stomach (gastroesophageal junction) move upward into the chest cavity through the weakened or enlarged esophageal hiatus. This type of hernia is often associated with gastroesophageal reflux disease (GERD) and can lead to symptoms such as heartburn, regurgitation, and chest pain.

In a sliding hiatal hernia, the gastroesophageal junction moves in and out of the chest cavity with changes in position, such as when a person lies down or stands up. While sliding hiatal hernias can be asymptomatic in some cases, they can cause discomfort and complications, making proper diagnosis and management essential.

2.2 Paraesophageal Hiatal Hernia

A paraesophageal hiatal hernia, also known as a type II hiatal hernia, is less common than a sliding hiatal hernia but potentially more serious. In this type of hernia, a portion of the stomach, often the greater curvature, herniates through the esophageal hiatus and into the chest cavity, alongside the esophagus. Unlike a sliding hernia, the gastroesophageal junction remains in its normal position.

Paraesophageal hernias are concerning because they can lead to complications such as gastric volvulus, a condition where the stomach rotates on its axis, potentially cutting off blood supply and causing severe pain and tissue damage. These hernias can also lead to obstructive symptoms, making swallowing difficult and uncomfortable. Surgical intervention is often recommended to repair paraesophageal hiatal hernias and prevent complications.

2.3 Mixed Hiatal Hernia

Mixed hiatal hernias, as the name suggests, combine characteristics of both sliding and paraesophageal hernias. In these cases, the gastroesophageal junction slides into the chest cavity, as seen in sliding hernias, and a portion of the stomach also herniates alongside the esophagus, similar to paraesophageal hernias.

Mixed hiatal hernias can be particularly challenging to diagnose and manage, as they present a combination of symptoms and potential complications from both types. These hernias often require surgical intervention to correct the anatomical abnormalities and reduce the risk of complications.

Understanding the distinctions between these types of hiatal hernias is essential for healthcare professionals to provide accurate diagnoses and determine the most appropriate treatment strategies. Each type carries its own set of symptoms, risks, and considerations, making it imperative to tailor management approaches to the specific type of hernia and the needs of the individual patient.

CHAPTER 3

Diagnosis

Diagnosing hiatal hernia syndrome is a crucial step in providing effective treatment and management for affected individuals. The diagnostic process typically involves a combination of medical history and physical examination, imaging and diagnostic tests, and the consideration of differential diagnoses to rule out other conditions with similar symptoms.

3.1 Medical History and Physical Examination

Medical History:

- Obtaining a detailed medical history is often the initial step in the diagnostic process. Healthcare professionals will inquire about the patient's symptoms, their duration, and any factors that exacerbate or alleviate the symptoms. A history of heartburn, regurgitation, chest pain, difficulty swallowing, or other related symptoms is essential information for diagnosis.

- Patients may be asked about their lifestyle and risk factors, such as obesity, smoking, or heavy lifting, as these factors can contribute to hiatal hernia development.

Physical Examination:

- During the physical examination, healthcare providers will typically focus on the abdominal and chest areas. They may perform palpation to assess for tenderness or discomfort in the upper abdomen and chest.

- Evaluation of respiratory and cardiovascular function may be conducted to rule out other potential causes of chest pain or shortness of breath.

3.2 Imaging and Diagnostic Tests

Imaging Studies:

- Imaging is a critical component of hiatal hernia diagnosis. Common imaging studies include:

    - **Barium swallow:** This involves swallowing a contrast material (barium) that is visible on X-rays. It helps visualize the movement of the esophagus and stomach and can reveal the presence and size of a hiatal hernia.

    - **Upper gastrointestinal endoscopy:** This procedure involves inserting a flexible, lighted tube (endoscope) through the mouth to examine the esophagus, stomach, and upper part of the small intestine. It can directly visualize the herniated portion of the stomach and assess for inflammation or other abnormalities.

Diagnostic Tests:

- Additional diagnostic tests may be used to assess the severity of gastroesophageal reflux disease (GERD) often associated with hiatal hernias. These tests may include:

  - **Esophageal pH monitoring:** This test measures the acidity in the esophagus over a 24-hour period, providing information about the extent of acid reflux.

- **Manometry:** Esophageal manometry measures the pressure and coordination of muscle contractions in the esophagus, helping to evaluate how well the esophagus functions.

3.3 Differential Diagnosis

Differential diagnosis is an essential aspect of the diagnostic process for hiatal hernia syndrome, as its symptoms can overlap with those of other conditions. Conditions that healthcare providers may consider in the differential diagnosis include:

- **Gastroesophageal reflux disease (GERD):** Hiatal hernias are often associated with GERD, but they can occur independently. Distinguishing between the two is crucial, as the treatment approaches may vary.

- **Angina or heart-related conditions:** Chest pain associated with hiatal hernias can mimic heart-related chest pain. It's essential to rule out cardiac causes through ECG, stress testing, and other cardiac evaluations.

- **Peptic ulcers:** The symptoms of peptic ulcers, such as epigastric pain, can resemble those of hiatal hernias. Endoscopy can help differentiate between the two conditions.

- **Esophageal motility disorders:** Conditions like achalasia or diffuse esophageal spasm may present with dysphagia and mimic hiatal hernia symptoms. Manometry can help distinguish between these conditions.

A comprehensive diagnostic approach, which includes a thorough medical history, physical examination, imaging studies, and consideration of potential differential diagnoses, is essential to accurately identify and differentiate hiatal hernia syndrome from other medical conditions with similar presentations. This allows for tailored and effective treatment planning.

CHAPTER 4

Treatment Options

Treatment for hiatal hernia syndrome aims to alleviate symptoms, prevent complications, and improve the patient's quality of life. The approach to treatment can vary based on the severity of symptoms, the type of hiatal hernia, and the individual's overall health.

4.1 Lifestyle and Dietary Changes

Lifestyle and dietary modifications can play a significant role in managing hiatal hernia symptoms. These changes are often recommended as the first line of treatment, especially for individuals with mild to moderate symptoms. Some of the key lifestyle and dietary recommendations include:

- **Dietary Modifications:** Patients are advised to avoid or limit foods and beverages that can trigger acid reflux, such as spicy foods, citrus fruits, carbonated beverages, and fatty or fried foods. Smaller, more frequent meals are often suggested to reduce pressure on the stomach and esophagus.

- **Weight Management:** For individuals who are overweight or obese, weight loss is recommended to reduce intra-abdominal pressure, which can contribute to herniation and reflux.

- **Elevating the Head of the Bed:** Raising the head of the bed by 6 to 8 inches can help prevent nighttime reflux symptoms by using gravity to keep stomach acid from flowing into the esophagus.

- **Avoiding Tight Clothing:** Wearing tight clothing, especially around the abdomen, can put pressure on the stomach and exacerbate symptoms. Loose-fitting clothing is preferable.

- **Posture and Body Mechanics:** Practicing good posture and using proper body mechanics when lifting objects can reduce abdominal pressure and the risk of hernia exacerbation.

- **Smoking Cessation:** Quitting smoking is advised, as smoking can contribute to reflux symptoms and may exacerbate hiatal hernia-related issues.

- **Stress Reduction:** Managing stress through relaxation techniques, such as deep breathing and meditation, may help reduce the frequency and intensity of symptoms.

4.2 Medications

Medications may be prescribed to manage symptoms associated with hiatal hernia syndrome, particularly gastroesophageal reflux disease (GERD). Some common medications used in the treatment of hiatal hernias include:

- **Antacids:** Over-the-counter antacids can help neutralize stomach acid and provide short-term relief from heartburn and acid reflux symptoms.

- **Proton Pump Inhibitors (PPIs):** PPIs, such as omeprazole and pantoprazole, are commonly used to reduce the production of stomach acid. They are effective in managing GERD and preventing acid-related complications.

- **H2 Blockers:** Histamine-2 (H2) receptor antagonists, like ranitidine or famotidine, decrease the production of stomach acid and can be used to manage symptoms of acid reflux.

- **Prokinetic Agents:** These medications help improve the movement and coordination of the esophagus and stomach muscles, reducing the frequency of reflux episodes.

- **Antiemetic Drugs:** In cases where nausea and vomiting are significant symptoms, antiemetic drugs may be prescribed to alleviate these symptoms.

The choice of medications and their duration of use will depend on the severity of symptoms and the patient's response to treatment. It's important for individuals to work closely with their healthcare providers to determine the most suitable medications and dosages for their specific needs.

In more severe cases or when conservative treatments fail to provide relief, surgical intervention may be necessary. This may involve repairing the hernia and addressing associated complications, such as fundoplication to treat severe GERD. The decision to proceed with surgery is typically made on a case-by-case basis, considering the patient's overall health and the potential benefits of surgical correction.

4.3 Alternative Therapies

In addition to conventional medical treatments and lifestyle modifications, some individuals with hiatal hernia syndrome may explore alternative therapies as complementary approaches to alleviate symptoms and improve their overall well-being. It's important to note that the efficacy of alternative therapies can vary, and they should be used in consultation with a healthcare provider. Here are some alternative therapies that some people with hiatal hernia syndrome may consider:

1. **Acupuncture:** Acupuncture is a traditional Chinese practice that involves the insertion of fine needles into specific points on the body to balance energy flow. Some individuals find that acupuncture can help with pain management and stress reduction.

2. **Chiropractic Care:** Chiropractic adjustments may be used to address musculoskeletal issues, including those related to the

diaphragm and spine. However, the effectiveness of chiropractic care for hiatal hernia is a topic of debate within the medical community, and it should be pursued with caution.

3. **Herbal Remedies:** Some herbs and herbal supplements, such as slippery elm, chamomile, or aloe vera, are believed to have soothing properties that may help relieve heartburn and gastrointestinal discomfort. Consultation with a healthcare provider is essential to ensure safety and avoid potential interactions with medications.

4. **Homeopathy:** Homeopathic remedies are based on the principle of "like cures like." Homeopaths may recommend specific remedies to address

individual symptoms, but the scientific evidence supporting their effectiveness for hiatal hernia is limited.

5. **Yoga and Breathing Exercises:** Gentle yoga poses and deep breathing exercises can promote relaxation, improve posture, and enhance diaphragmatic function. These practices may help alleviate some symptoms and reduce stress.

6. **Dietary Supplements:** Certain dietary supplements, such as melatonin, may be used to manage symptoms of gastroesophageal reflux disease (GERD). However, the use of supplements should be discussed with a healthcare

provider to ensure safety and efficacy.

7. **Nutritional and Dietary Counseling:** Working with a registered dietitian or nutritionist can help individuals with hiatal hernias identify specific dietary triggers and develop customized meal plans that reduce the risk of reflux and discomfort.

It's crucial to approach alternative therapies with caution and in conjunction with conventional medical treatments. Hiatal hernia syndrome can lead to complications, and medical guidance is essential to monitor the condition and ensure the most appropriate and effective interventions. Moreover, individuals should be aware that the effectiveness of alternative therapies can vary from person to person, and what works for one individual may not work for another. Always consult with a qualified healthcare provider before pursuing alternative therapies to address hiatal hernia symptoms.

CHAPTER 5

Complications

Hiatal hernia syndrome can lead to a range of complications, some of which can be quite serious. These complications can result from the displacement of the stomach and the disruption of the normal function of the gastroesophageal junction. Here are three common complications associated with hiatal hernia syndrome:

5.1 Gastroesophageal Reflux Disease (GERD)

Gastroesophageal reflux disease (GERD) is a prevalent complication of hiatal hernia syndrome. When the stomach protrudes through the diaphragmatic opening into the chest cavity, the lower esophageal sphincter, which normally prevents stomach acid from flowing back into the esophagus, becomes compromised. As a result, individuals with hiatal hernias are at an increased risk of experiencing frequent and severe acid reflux.

GERD can lead to a variety of symptoms, including heartburn, regurgitation, chest pain, and difficulty swallowing. Over time, chronic acid reflux can cause inflammation and damage to the esophageal lining. If left untreated, it can lead to more severe complications, including esophagitis, esophageal strictures, and even an increased risk of esophageal cancer.

5.2 Barrett's Esophagus

Barrett's esophagus is a condition in which the normal squamous lining of the lower esophagus is replaced by specialized columnar epithelium, a type of tissue more resistant to stomach acid. It is considered a precancerous condition and is often associated with long-term, severe GERD, a common consequence of hiatal hernia syndrome.

The risk of developing esophageal adenocarcinoma, a form of esophageal cancer, significantly increases in individuals with Barrett's esophagus. Regular surveillance and monitoring through endoscopy and biopsies are recommended to detect early changes in the esophageal lining and initiate preventive measures or early treatment.

5.3 Strangulated Hiatal Hernia

A strangulated hiatal hernia is a severe and potentially life-threatening complication. In this condition, a portion of the stomach becomes trapped within the hiatal opening in the diaphragm, cutting off its blood supply. This can lead to tissue ischemia (lack of blood flow) and necrosis (tissue death).

Symptoms of a strangulated hiatal hernia may include severe chest pain, abdominal pain, nausea, vomiting, and difficulty swallowing. This condition is a medical emergency, and prompt surgical intervention is required to release the entrapped stomach and restore blood flow.

A strangulated hiatal hernia represents one of the most critical complications of hiatal hernia syndrome and necessitates immediate medical attention.

It's essential for individuals with hiatal hernia syndrome to be aware of these potential complications and to seek timely medical evaluation and appropriate management. Regular monitoring and adherence to treatment recommendations can help mitigate the risks associated with these complications and improve the overall prognosis for individuals with hiatal hernia syndrome.

CHAPTER 6

Living with Hiatal Hernia

Living with a hiatal hernia, especially when experiencing symptoms, can be challenging. However, by making certain adjustments to your lifestyle, diet, and daily habits, you can manage the condition effectively.

6.1 Diet and Nutrition

Diet and nutrition play a significant role in managing hiatal hernia symptoms, particularly those related to gastroesophageal reflux. Here are some dietary guidelines to consider:

- **Avoid Trigger Foods:** Identify and avoid foods and beverages that trigger acid reflux and heartburn. Common triggers include spicy foods, citrus fruits, tomatoes, chocolate, caffeine, and fatty or fried foods.

- **Smaller, Frequent Meals:** Instead of three large meals, opt for smaller, more frequent meals to reduce pressure on the stomach and minimize the risk of reflux. This can also help with weight management.

- **Chew Thoroughly:** Take your time to chew your food thoroughly, as this can reduce the risk of swallowing air, which can lead to bloating.

- **Stay Hydrated:** Ensure you stay well-hydrated throughout the day by drinking water. However, avoid drinking large amounts of fluids during meals, as this can increase stomach pressure.

- **Acidic and Alkaline Foods:** Some individuals find that consuming alkaline foods, such as certain fruits and vegetables, can help balance stomach acidity. Discuss this with your healthcare provider.

- **Elevate the Head of the Bed:** If nighttime reflux is a concern,

raise the head of your bed by 6
to 8 inches using blocks or bed
risers to keep stomach acid
from flowing into the
esophagus.

- **Avoid Lying Down After Meals:** Wait at least two to three hours after eating before lying down or going to bed to reduce the risk of reflux.

- **Maintain a Food Diary:** Keeping a food diary can help you identify specific trigger foods and patterns that worsen your symptoms.

6.2 Coping with Symptoms

Managing hiatal hernia symptoms can greatly improve your quality of life.

Here are strategies to help cope with these symptoms:

- **Medications:** If prescribed by your healthcare provider, take medications such as antacids, proton pump inhibitors (PPIs), or H2 blockers as directed to control acid reflux and heartburn.

- **Posture and Body Mechanics:** Be mindful of your posture and body mechanics, especially when lifting heavy objects. Using proper body mechanics can reduce pressure on the abdomen and minimize the risk of herniation.

- **Stress Reduction:** Stress can exacerbate symptoms, so engage in stress-reduction techniques like deep breathing, meditation, or yoga to promote relaxation.

- **Wear Loose-Fitting Clothing:** Opt for loose-fitting clothing, especially around the waist, to reduce pressure on the stomach and diaphragm.

- **Elevate the Head While Sleeping:** As mentioned earlier, raising the head of your bed can help alleviate nighttime reflux symptoms.

- **Regular Exercise:** Engage in regular, moderate exercise to help with weight management and overall well-being. Consult your healthcare provider for exercise recommendations that are safe and appropriate for your condition.

- **Support and Education:**
  Consider joining support
  groups or seeking educational
  resources to connect with
  others who have hiatal hernias
  and to learn more about
  managing the condition.

Living with a hiatal hernia may
require ongoing management and
adaptation, but by making these
changes and working closely with
your healthcare provider, you can
effectively manage your symptoms
and lead a comfortable and fulfilling
life. If your symptoms worsen or if
you experience new or severe
complications, consult your
healthcare provider for further
evaluation and treatment options.

6.3 Preventative Measures

Preventative measures can help reduce the risk of developing hiatal hernias, alleviate symptoms, and minimize the chances of complications. While not all factors leading to hiatal hernias can be controlled, there are steps you can take to promote a healthier lifestyle and potentially prevent or manage the condition more effectively:

1. **Maintain a Healthy Weight:** Obesity and excess abdominal fat can increase intra-abdominal pressure, which may contribute to the development or exacerbation of hiatal hernias. Adopt a well-balanced diet and engage in regular physical activity to achieve and maintain a healthy weight.

2. **Dietary Awareness:** Be
    conscious of your diet and its
    impact on acid reflux. Avoid
    trigger foods and beverages,
    and consider adopting a more
    plant-based and alkaline diet if
    you find it helps reduce your
    symptoms.

3. **Portion Control:** Eating
    smaller, more frequent meals
    rather than large, heavy meals
    can reduce the pressure on your
    stomach and lower esophagus,
    potentially preventing or
    alleviating symptoms.

4. **Posture and Lifting
    Techniques:** Maintain good
    posture and use proper body
    mechanics when lifting heavy
    objects to reduce the risk of
    abdominal strain, which can
    contribute to hiatal hernias.

5. **Smoking Cessation:** If you are a smoker, quitting smoking is advisable. Smoking can weaken the lower esophageal sphincter, contributing to acid reflux.

6. **Stress Reduction:** Chronic stress can worsen gastrointestinal symptoms, including those related to hiatal hernias. Engage in stress-reduction techniques like relaxation exercises, meditation, and mindfulness to manage stress effectively.

7. **Wear Loose-Fitting Clothing:** Opt for comfortable, loose-fitting clothing, particularly around the waist, to minimize abdominal pressure.

8. **Elevate the Head of the Bed:** If you have frequent nighttime

reflux, consider elevating the head of your bed by 6 to 8 inches to use gravity to prevent acid reflux.

9. **Regular Check-Ups:** If you have a hiatal hernia or are at risk due to family history or other factors, schedule regular check-ups with your healthcare provider to monitor your condition and discuss any necessary adjustments to your treatment plan.

10. **Consult a Registered Dietitian:** Working with a registered dietitian can help you develop a personalized meal plan that takes into account your dietary preferences and specific trigger foods.

11. **Avoid Large Meals Before Bed:** To reduce nighttime reflux, avoid consuming large meals shortly before bedtime, and allow several hours between eating and lying down.

12. **Follow Medical Recommendations:** If you have been diagnosed with a hiatal hernia or gastroesophageal reflux disease (GERD), adhere to the treatment plan and medication regimen recommended by your healthcare provider.

While these preventative measures can contribute to managing hiatal hernias and their associated symptoms, it's essential to remember that not all hiatal hernias can be prevented, as some may have a genetic or congenital basis. If you experience severe or persistent symptoms or complications, consult your healthcare provider for an accurate diagnosis and appropriate treatment.

CHAPTER 7

Recovery and Aftercare

Recovery and aftercare play a crucial role in the management of hiatal hernia, particularly after surgical intervention. Following surgical repair, patients must take steps to ensure a smooth recovery and minimize the risk of complications.

7.1 Postoperative Care

After hiatal hernia surgery, whether it's a laparoscopic or open procedure, postoperative care is vital for a successful recovery. Here are some key aspects of postoperative care:

1. **Hospital Stay:** The length of your hospital stay will depend on the type of surgery, your overall health, and the surgeon's recommendations. For laparoscopic procedures, a shorter hospital stay is common, often a day or less. For open surgeries, the stay may be longer.

2. **Pain Management:** Pain and discomfort are typical after surgery. Your healthcare team will provide pain management strategies, which may include medication or other pain relief techniques.

3. **Dietary Progression:** You'll typically start with a clear liquid diet and then progress to a soft diet as you tolerate it. The goal is to gradually reintroduce solid foods. Follow the dietary instructions provided by your healthcare team.

4. **Medications:** Continue taking any prescribed medications, such as proton pump inhibitors or other acid-reducing drugs, as directed by your surgeon. These medications help prevent reflux and promote healing.

5. **Avoid Straining:** Refrain from heavy lifting or strenuous physical activity during the early stages of recovery, as this can strain the surgical site.

6. **Follow-Up Appointments:**
Attend all scheduled follow-up
appointments with your
surgeon to monitor your
progress and discuss any
concerns or issues. These
appointments are crucial for
ensuring that your recovery is
on track.

7. **Incision Care:** If you have
open surgery, it's essential to
keep the incision site clean and
dry to prevent infection. Follow
any wound care instructions
provided by your healthcare
team.

8. **Gradual Return to Normal
Activities:** As you recover,
gradually resume normal
activities as advised by your
surgeon. You should avoid

intense physical exertion for some time.

9. **Dietary Modifications:** After surgery, you may need to make long-term dietary modifications to reduce the risk of reflux and discomfort. Your surgeon or a registered dietitian can provide guidance on an appropriate diet plan.

10. **Monitor for Complications:** Be vigilant for any signs of complications, such as infection, bleeding, or difficulty swallowing. If you experience any unusual symptoms, contact your healthcare provider promptly.

11. **Recovery Timeline:** The duration of your recovery will vary depending on the surgical

approach and your individual
response to the procedure. Your
healthcare team will provide
you with an estimated timeline
for returning to your regular
activities.

12. **Lifestyle Modifications:**
Continue with lifestyle
modifications that were
recommended before surgery,
such as weight management,
stress reduction, and posture
improvement, to reduce the risk
of recurrent hiatal hernias.

It's important to maintain open
communication with your healthcare
provider throughout the recovery
process. They can address any
concerns, adjust your treatment plan
as needed, and ensure that you are on
the path to optimal recovery. With
proper postoperative care and

adherence to recommendations, most
individuals can experience significant
relief from hiatal hernia symptoms
and enjoy an improved quality of life.

7.2 Managing Pain and Discomfort

Managing pain and discomfort is a
crucial aspect of the recovery process
for individuals with hiatal hernia,
particularly after surgical
intervention. Here are some strategies
to help alleviate pain and discomfort
during recovery:

1. **Pain Medication:** Follow your
   healthcare provider's
   instructions regarding pain
   medication. Over-the-counter
   pain relievers, such as
   acetaminophen or non-steroidal

anti-inflammatory drugs
(NSAIDs), may be
recommended. Stronger
prescription pain medications
may be prescribed after
surgery. Take them as directed
to manage pain effectively.

2. **Positioning:** Find a
    comfortable and supportive
    position that minimizes strain
    on the surgical area. Elevating
    your upper body with pillows,
    especially while sleeping, can
    help reduce nighttime reflux
    symptoms and alleviate
    discomfort.

3. **Breathing Exercises:** Deep
    breathing exercises can help
    prevent lung complications and
    reduce postoperative pain.
    Regular deep breaths and gentle

coughing can help maintain lung function.

4. **Walking and Gentle Movement:** Encourage gentle movement and walking as soon as your healthcare provider approves. This can help prevent complications, improve circulation, and reduce stiffness.

5. **Ice Packs:** Applying ice packs to the surgical area can help reduce swelling and provide temporary relief from pain. Be sure to use a barrier, such as a cloth, between the ice pack and your skin to avoid frostbite.

6. **Dietary Modifications:** Follow your prescribed diet plan, which may include clear liquids, soft foods, and a

gradual progression to solid foods. This can help prevent postoperative nausea, vomiting, and discomfort.

7. **Hydration:** Stay well-hydrated, as dehydration can exacerbate postoperative discomfort. Sip on clear fluids and follow the dietary guidelines provided by your healthcare team.

8. **Avoid Straining:** Avoid heavy lifting or any activities that place excessive strain on the surgical area, as this can lead to increased discomfort or complications.

9. **Posture and Body Mechanics:** Be mindful of your posture and use proper body mechanics when moving or getting up.

Good posture can reduce pressure on the abdomen and improve comfort.

10. **Stool Softeners:** Pain medications can sometimes cause constipation. If this is a concern, ask your healthcare provider about the use of stool softeners or mild laxatives to prevent discomfort during bowel movements.

11. **Follow Healthcare Provider's Instructions:** Always follow the specific postoperative care instructions provided by your healthcare provider. These may include wound care, medication schedules, and restrictions on certain activities.

12. **Communicate with Your Healthcare Team:** If you

experience severe or persistent pain, or if you have concerns about your recovery, don't hesitate to communicate with your healthcare team. They can adjust your pain management plan or provide additional guidance to enhance your comfort.

Pain and discomfort are common during the recovery period after hiatal hernia surgery, but they should gradually subside over time. It's important to remember that everyone's recovery experience is unique, and some discomfort is expected. By following your healthcare provider's guidance and adhering to these strategies, you can effectively manage pain and discomfort during your recovery process.

7.3 Long-Term Outlook

The long-term outlook for individuals with hiatal hernia depends on several factors, including the type of hernia, the presence of complications, the success of treatment, and lifestyle management. Here are some considerations for the long-term outlook:

1. **Type of Hiatal Hernia:** The type of hiatal hernia you have can influence your long-term prognosis. Sliding hiatal hernias are generally more common and may have different outcomes compared to paraesophageal or mixed hiatal hernias.

2. **Complications:** If you have experienced complications like

gastroesophageal reflux disease (GERD), Barrett's esophagus, or a strangulated hiatal hernia, ongoing management and monitoring are essential. The prognosis may vary based on the severity of these complications.

3. **Treatment Success:** The success of treatment, whether through lifestyle modifications, medications, or surgery, can significantly impact your long-term outlook. Successful management of symptoms and complications can lead to an improved quality of life.

4. **Lifestyle Modifications:** Long-term adherence to lifestyle modifications, including dietary changes, weight management, stress reduction, and good

posture, can help minimize the risk of symptom recurrence and complications.

5. **Medication Management:** If you are prescribed medications, such as proton pump inhibitors (PPIs) or other acid-reducing drugs, it's important to follow your healthcare provider's recommendations for their long-term use.

6. **Dietary Considerations:** A long-term dietary plan that avoids trigger foods and promotes overall gastrointestinal health can help prevent reflux and related symptoms.

7. **Regular Check-Ups:** Routine follow-up appointments with your healthcare provider are

crucial for monitoring your condition and addressing any changes or concerns.

8. **Complications Surveillance:** For individuals with complications like Barrett's esophagus, regular surveillance through endoscopy and biopsies is necessary to detect early changes and initiate preventive measures.

9. **Weight Management:** If obesity contributed to your hiatal hernia, maintaining a healthy weight can significantly improve your long-term outlook and minimize the risk of recurrence.

10. **Stress Management:** Continued stress reduction techniques and practices can

help prevent exacerbation of symptoms and maintain overall well-being.

11. **Hydration:** Staying well-hydrated can promote healthy digestion and reduce the risk of reflux symptoms.

12. **Adaptation to Changing Needs:** Over time, your healthcare needs may change, so it's important to adapt your management plan accordingly. This may involve medication adjustments, dietary changes, or additional interventions.

Appropriate management and ongoing care, many individuals with hiatal hernias can enjoy a good long-term quality of life. However, it's important to remain vigilant and continue working closely with your healthcare provider to address any changes in your condition and to ensure the best possible outcome over the years.

7.4 Ongoing Research in Hiatal Hernia Syndrome

Hiatal Hernia Syndrome (HHS) is a medical condition characterized by the protrusion of a portion of the stomach into the chest cavity through the esophageal hiatus in the diaphragm. Ongoing research in HHS is vital to better understand the condition, improve diagnostic techniques, optimize treatment strategies, and enhance patients' quality of life. Some key areas of ongoing research in HHS include:

1. Genetics and Risk Factors:

- Researchers have been exploring genetic factors that might predispose individuals to HHS. Understanding the genetic basis of the condition could help identify at-risk populations and develop personalized treatment approaches.

2. Biomarkers and Diagnostics:

- Advancements in medical imaging and biomarker identification are of significant interest. Researchers are working on developing non-invasive diagnostic tests and imaging techniques to detect and classify hiatal hernias more accurately and efficiently. This can help in early diagnosis and intervention.

3. Minimally Invasive Surgical Techniques:

- The field of surgery is seeing rapid advancements in minimally invasive techniques such as laparoscopy and robotic-assisted surgery. Ongoing research focuses on refining these procedures for hiatal hernia repair, which can lead to shorter recovery times and reduced postoperative pain.

4. Improved Postoperative Outcomes:

- Researchers are exploring ways to enhance postoperative outcomes, reduce complications, and improve the long-term success of hiatal hernia repairs. This includes studying techniques to prevent

hernia recurrence and manage
complications like
gastroesophageal reflux disease
(GERD).

5. Medical Management:

- The development of more
  effective medications for
  managing symptoms of hiatal
  hernia and related conditions
  like GERD is an ongoing area
  of research. New drug therapies
  may offer better relief and
  fewer side effects for patients.

6. Predictive Modeling and Risk Assessment:

- Computational approaches and
  predictive modeling are being
  used to assess an individual's
  risk of developing HHS and
  predict the likelihood of
  complications. These models

can assist in early intervention and personalized treatment planning.

7. Patient Outcomes and Quality of Life:

- Research is increasingly focusing on assessing the impact of HHS and its treatments on patients' quality of life. This involves patient-reported outcomes, psychological well-being, and long-term follow-up studies to understand the holistic effects of the condition and its management.

8. Regenerative Medicine and Tissue Engineering:

- In regenerative medicine, there is ongoing research into developing tissue engineering techniques to repair the damaged diaphragmatic tissue, potentially offering new ways to treat hiatal hernias. These approaches aim to restore normal anatomy and function.

9. Advances in Endoscopy:

- Endoscopic procedures, such as endoluminal fundoplication, are being investigated as less invasive alternatives for hiatal hernia repair. These procedures may offer advantages in terms of recovery and patient comfort.

10. Epidemiology and Healthcare Policy:

- Understanding the prevalence and economic burden of HHS is important for shaping healthcare policies and resource allocation. Ongoing epidemiological studies help identify at-risk populations and prioritize research and treatment efforts.

Ongoing research in Hiatal Hernia Syndrome encompasses a wide range of areas, from understanding genetic and risk factors to improving diagnostics, surgical techniques, postoperative outcomes, and patient quality of life. Advances in regenerative medicine and the development of minimally invasive procedures hold promise for the future, offering potential benefits for patients suffering from this condition. It's essential to stay updated with the latest research findings and developments in HHS to provide the best care and treatment options for affected individuals.